WOOD PELLET SMOKER AND GRILL COOKBOOK

Delicious recipes with real BBQ flavor for beginners and advanced users of the grill.

STEVE MC LEAN

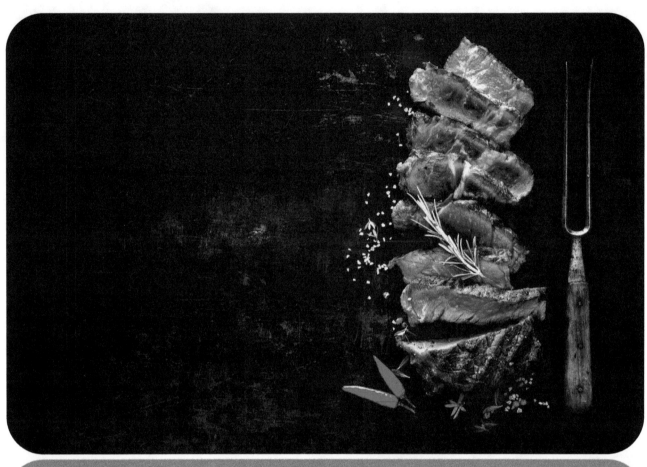

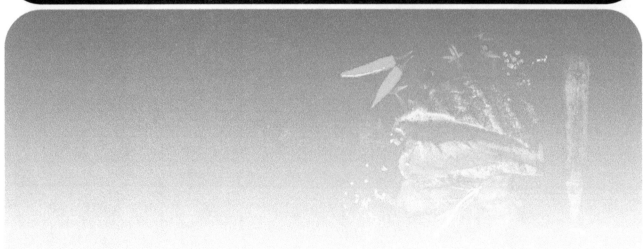

1. Perfect Beef Tenderloin

Prep Time: 10 minutes | Cooking Time: 1 hour 19 minutes | Temperature: 250F| Servings: 12

Ingredients:

o 1 (5-lb.) beef tenderloin, trimmed
o Kosher salt, to taste
o ¼ cup olive oil
o Ground black pepper, to taste

Directions:

1. Tie the tenderloin with kitchen strings at 7 to 8 places.
2. Season tenderloin with salt generously.
3. Cover the tenderloin with a plastic wrap and set aside at room temperature for 1 hour.
4. Preheat the Traeger Grill at 250F with a closed lid for 15 minutes.
5. Now, coat the tenderloin with oil and season with black pepper.
6. Arrange tenderloin onto the grill and cook for 55 to 65 minutes.
7. Now, place cooking grate directly over hot coals and sear tenderloin for 2 minutes per side.
8. Remove the tenderloin and rest for 10 minutes.
9. Slice and serve.

NUTRITION:

Calories: 425|Fat:21.5g | Carb: 0g| Protein:54.7g

2. Versatile Beef Tenderloin

Prep Time: 15 minutes | Cooking Time: 2 hours 5 minutes | Temperature: 230F| Servings: 6

Ingredients:

For Brandy Butter

- ½ cup butter
- 1 oz. brandy

For Brandy Sauce:

- 2 oz. brandy
- 8 garlic cloves, minced
- ¼ cup mixed fresh herbs (parsley, rosemary, and thyme), chopped

- 2 tsp. honey
- 2 tsp. hot English mustard

For Tenderloin:

- 1 (2-lb.) center-cut beef tenderloin
- Salt and cracked black peppercorns, to taste

Directions:

1. Set the temperature of Traeger Grill to 230F and preheat with a closed lid for 15 minutes.
2. For brandy butter: in a pan, melt butter, then stir in brandy and remove from heat. Cover and set aside. Keep warm.
3. For brandy sauce: in a bowl, add all the ingredients and mix well.
4. Season tenderloin with salt and black peppercorns generously.
5. Coat tenderloin with brandy sauce evenly.

6. With a baster-injector, inject tenderloin with brandy butter.

7. Place the tenderloin onto the grill and cook for 1 ½ to 2 hours. Injecting with brandy butter occasionally.

8. Remove the tenderloin from the grill and rest for 10 minutes.

9. Slice and serve.

NUTRITION:

Calories: 496|Fat: 29.3g| Carb: 4.4g | Protein:44.4g

3. Buttered Tenderloin

Prep Time: 10 minutes| Cooking Time: 45 minutes| Temperature: 300F| Servings:8

Ingredients:

- o 1 (4-lb.) beef tenderloin, trimmed
- o Cracked black pepper and smoked salt, to taste
- o 3 tbsp. butter, melted

Directions:

1. Set the temperature of Traeger Grill to 300F and preheat with a closed lid for 15 minutes.
2. Season the tenderloin with salt and pepper, and then rub with butter.
3. Place the tenderloin onto the grill and cook for 45 minutes.
4. Remove the tenderloin from the grill and rest for 10 minutes.
5. Slice and serve.

NUTRITION:

Calories: 505|Fat: 25.1g | Carb: 0g| Protein: 65.7g

4. Delish Beef Brisket

Prep Time: 10 minutes | Cooking Time: 7 hours | Temperature: 250F|
Servings:10

Ingredients:

- 1 cup paprika
- ¾ cup sugar
- 3 tbsp. garlic salt
- 3 tbsp. onion powder
- 1 tbsp. celery salt
- 1 tbsp. lemon pepper
- 1 tbsp. ground black pepper
- 1 tsp. cayenne pepper
- 1 tsp. mustard powder
- ½ tsp. dried thyme, crushed
- 1 (5-6-lb.) beef brisket, trimmed

Directions:

1. Place all ingredients in a bowl, except for beef brisket, and mix well.
2. Rub the brisket with spice mixture.
3. Cover the brisket with a plastic wrap and refrigerate overnight.
4. Set the temperature of Traeger Grill to 250F and preheat with a closed lid for 15 minutes.
5. Place the brisket onto the grill over indirect heat and cook for 3 to 3 ½ hours.
6. Flip and cook for 3 to 3 ½ hours more.
7. Remove the brisket from the grill and rest for 10 minutes.
8. Slice and serve.

NUTRITION:

Calories: 536|Fat: 15.6g| Carb: 24.8g| Protein: 71.1g

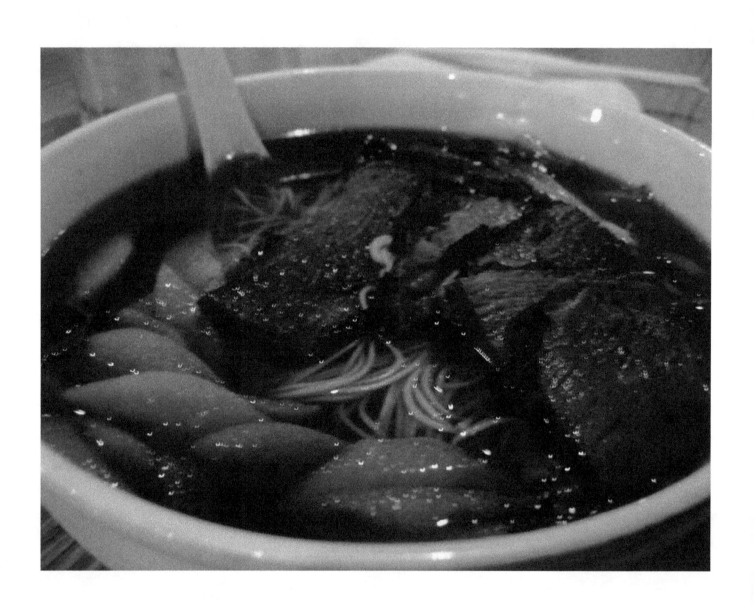

5. St. Patrick Day's Corned Beef

Prep Time: 15 minutes | Cooking Time: 7 hours | Temperature: 275F|
Servings:14

Ingredients:

- 6 lb. corned beef brisket, drained, rinsed and pat dried
- Ground black pepper, to taste
- 8 oz. light beer

Directions:

1. Set the temperature of Traeger Grill to 275F and preheat with a closed lid for 15 minutes.
2. Sprinkle the beef brisket with the spice packet evenly.
3. Place the brisket onto the grill and cook for 3 to 4 hours.
4. Remove from grill and transfer briskets into an aluminum pan.
5. Add enough beer just to cover the bottom of the pan.
6. Cover the pan with a piece of foil, leaving one corner open to let out steam.
7. Cook for 2 to 3 hours.
8. Remove the brisket from the grill and rest for 10 minutes.
9. Slice and serve.

NUTRITION:

Calories: 337|Fat: 24.3g| Carb: 0.6g| Protein: 26.1g

6. Spiced Rump Roast

Prep Time: 10 minutes| Cooking Time: 6 hours | Temperature: 200F|
Servings: 8

Ingredients:

- 1 tsp. smoked paprika
- 1 tsp. cayenne pepper
- 1 tsp. onion powder
- 1 tsp. garlic powder
- Salt and ground black pepper, to taste
- 3 lb. beef rump roast
- ¼ cup Worcestershire sauce

Directions:

1. Set the temperature of Traeger Grill to 200F and preheat with closed lid for 15 minutes, using charcoal.
2. Mix together all the spices in a bowl.
3. Coat the rump roast with Worcestershire sauce evenly and then rub with spice mixture generously.
4. Place the rump roast onto the grill and cook for 5 to 6 hours.
5. Remove the roast from the grill and rest for 10 minutes.
6. Slice and serve.

NUTRITION:

Calories: 252|Fat: 9.1g| Carb: 2.3g| Protein: 37.8g

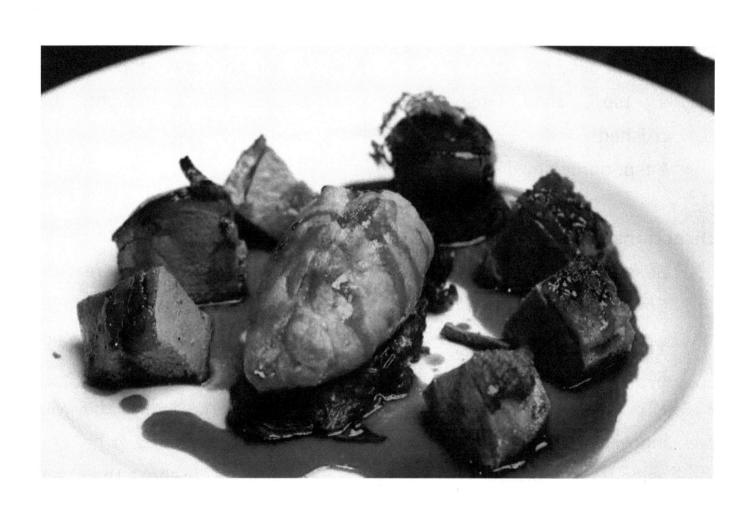

7. Prime Rib Roast

Prep Time: 10 minutes | Cooking Time: 3 hours 50 minutes | Temperature: 230F | Servings: 10

Ingredients:

- 1 (5-lb.) prime rib roast
- Salt, to taste
- 5 tbsp. olive oil
- 4 tsp. dried rosemary, crushed
- 2 tsp. garlic powder
- 1 tsp. onion powder
- 1 tsp. paprika
- ½ tsp. cayenne pepper
- Ground black pepper, to taste

Directions:

1. Season the roast with salt.
2. Cover the roast with a plastic wrap and refrigerate for 24 hours.
3. Mix together the remaining ingredients in a bowl and set aside for 1 hour.
4. Rub the roast with oil mixture.
5. Arrange the roast in a baking sheet and refrigerate for 6 to 12 hours.
6. Set the temperature of Traeger Grill to 225 to 230F and preheat with a closed lid for 15 minutes.
7. Place the roast onto the grill and cook for 3 to 3 ½ hours.
8. Meanwhile, preheat the oven to 500F.
9. Remove the roast from the grill and place onto a baking sheet.
10. Bake the roast in the oven for 15 to 20 minutes.

11. Remove the roast and rest for 10 minutes.

12. Slice and serve.

NUTRITION:

Calories: 605|Fat:47.6g | Carb: 3.8g| Protein: 38g

8. Real Treat Chuck Roast

Prep Time: 10 minutes | Cooking Time: 4 ½ hours | Temperature: 250F|
Servings: 8

Ingredients:

- 2 tbsp. onion powder
- 2 tbsp. garlic powder
- 1 tbsp. red chili powder
- 1 tbsp. cayenne pepper
- Salt and ground black pepper, to taste
- 1 (3 lb.) beef chuck roast
- 16 fluid oz. warm beef broth

Directions:

1. Set the temperature of Traeger Grill to 250F and preheat with a closed lid for 15 minutes.
2. In a bowl, mix together spices, salt, and black pepper.
3. Rub the chuck roast with spice mixture.
4. Place the rump roast onto the grill and cook for 1 ½ hour per side.
5. Now, arrange the chuck roast in a steaming pan with beef broth.
6. With a piece of foil, cover the pan and cook for 2 to 3 hours.
7. Remove the chuck roast from the grill and rest for 20 minutes.
8. Slice and serve.

NUTRITION:

Calories: 645 |Fat: 48g| Carb: 4.2g| Protein: 46.4g

9. Tri-Tip Roast

Prep Time: 10 minutes| Cooking Time: 35 minutes| Temperature: 250F & 400F| Servings: 8

Ingredients:

o 1 tbsp. granulated onion

o 1 tbsp. granulated garlic

o Salt and ground black pepper, to taste

o 1 (3-lb.) tri-tip roast, trimmed

Directions:

1. In a bowl, add all ingredients except for the roast and mix well.

2. Coat the roast with spice mixture. Set aside until grill heats.

3. Set the temperature of Traeger Grill to 250F and preheat with a closed lid for 15 minutes.

4. Place the roast onto the grill and cook for 25 minutes.

5. Now, set the grill to 350 to 400F and preheat with a closed lid for 15 minutes. Sear roast for 3 to 5 minutes per side.

6. Remove the roast and rest for 20 minutes.

7. Slice and serve.

NUTRITION:

Calories: 313|Fat: 14.2g| Carb: 0.8g| Protein: 45.7g

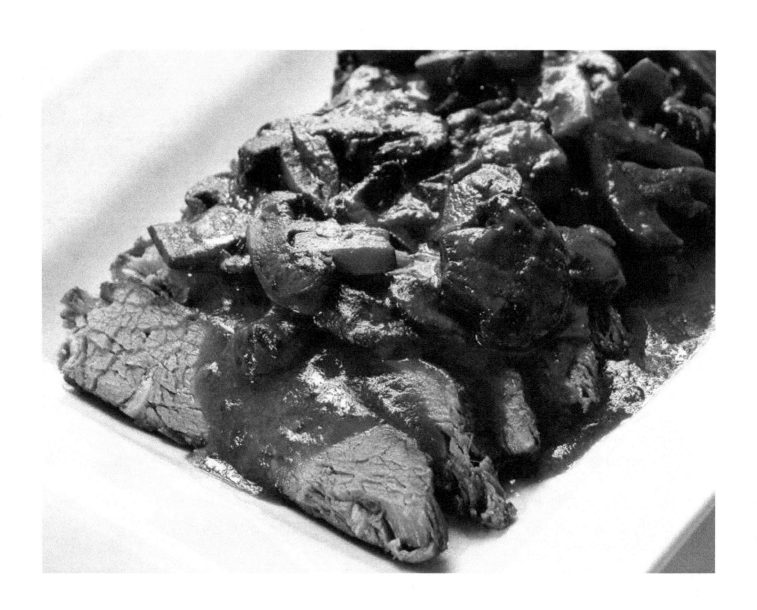

10. Flank Steak

Prep Time: 15 minutes | Cooking Time: 30 minutes | Temperature: 225F| Servings: 6

Ingredients:

- o   1 (2-lb.) beef flank steak
- o   2 tbsp. olive oil
- o   ¼ cup BBQ rub
- o   2 tbsp. butter, melted

Directions:

1. Set the temperature of Traeger Grill to 225F and preheat with a closed lid for 15 minutes.
2. Coat the steak with oil and season with BBQ rub.
3. Place the steak onto the grill and cook for 10 to 15 minutes per side.
4. Remove the steak from the grill and rest for 10 minutes.
5. Slice and drizzle with melted butter. Serve.

NUTRITION:

Calories: 355|Fat: 17.9g| Carb: 0g| Protein: 45.9g

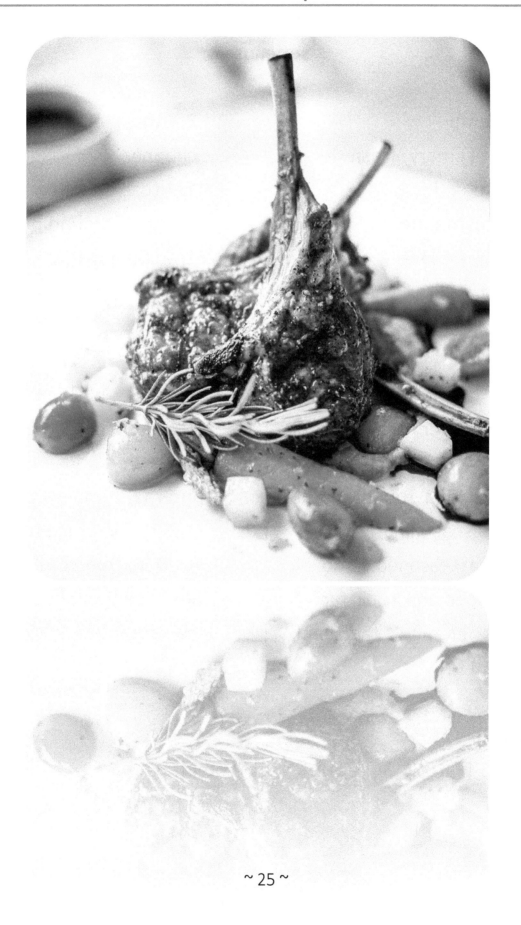

11. Traeger Smoked Lamb Chops

Prep Time: 10 minutes | Cooking Time: 50 minutes | Temperature: 225F | Servings: 4

Ingredients:

- 1 rack lamb
- 2 tbsp rosemary, fresh
- 2 tbsp sage, fresh
- 1 tbsp thyme, fresh
- 2 garlic cloves, roughly chopped
- 2 tbsp shallots, roughly chopped
- 1/2 tbsp salt
- 1/2 tbsp ground pepper
- 1/4 cup olive oil
- 1 tbsp honey

Directions:

1. Preheat the Traeger to 225F.
2. Combine everything except for the lamb in a food processor and rub the lamb with this seasoning.
3. Place the seasoned lamb on the Traeger and cook for 45 minutes or until the lamb reaches 120F.
4. Sear the lamb on the Traeger for 2 minutes per side or until the lamb's internal temperature reaches 125F for medium-rare or 145F for medium.
5. Rest for 5 minutes, slice, and serve.

NUTRITION:

Calories: 916 |Fat: 78.3g| Carb: 2.7g| Protein: 47g

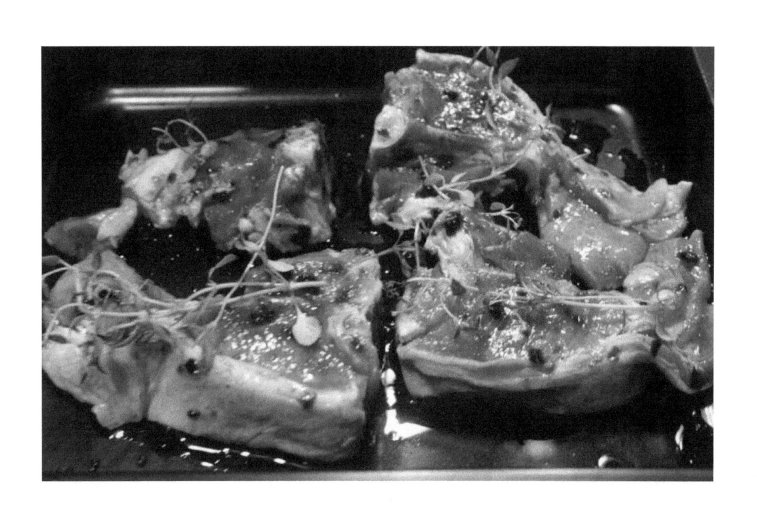

12. Traeger Smoked Lamb Shoulder

Prep Time: 20 minutes | Cooking Time: 3 hours| Temperature: 225F|
Servings: 7

Ingredients:

- 5 lb. lamb shoulder
- 1 cup cider vinegar
- 2 tbsp. oil
- 2 tbsp. kosher salt
- 2 tbsp. black pepper, freshly ground
- 1 tbsp. dried rosemary

For the Spritz
- 1 cup apple cider vinegar
- 1 cup apple juice

Directions:

1. Preheat the Traeger to 225F with a pan of water for moisture.
2. Trim excess fat from the lamb and rinse the meat with cold water. Pat dry.
3. Inject the cider vinegar in the meat, then pat dry with a clean paper towel.
4. Rub the meat with oil, salt, black pepper, and dried rosemary. Tie the lamb shoulder with a twine.
5. Place in the smoker for an hour, then spritz after every 15 minutes until the internal temperature reaches 165F.
6. Remove and rest for 1 hour. Slice and serve.

NUTRITION:

Calories: 472|Fat: 37g| Carb: 3g| Protein: 31g

13. Traeger Smoked Pulled Lamb Sliders

Prep Time: 10 minutes | Cooking Time: 9 hours| Temperature: 225F|
Servings: 7

Ingredients:

- 5 lb. lamb shoulder, boneless
- 1/2 cup olive oil
- 1/3 cup kosher salt
- 1/3 cup pepper, coarsely ground
- 1/3 cup granulated garlic

For the spritz
- 4 oz Worcestershire sauce
- 6 oz apple cider vinegar

Directions:

1. Preheat the Traeger to 225F with a pan of water for moisture.
2. Pat dry the lamb and rub with oil, salt, pepper, and garlic.
3. Place the lamb in the Traeger smoker for 90 minutes, then spritz every 30 minutes until the internal temperature reaches 165F.
4. Transfer the lamb to a foil pan, then add the remaining spritz liquid. Cover with a foil and place back in the Traeger.
5. Smoke until the internal temperature reaches 205F.
6. Remove from the smoker and rest for 30 minutes.
7. Slice and serve.

NUTRITION:

Calories: 235|Fat: 6g| Carb: 22g| Protein: 20g

14. Traeger Smoked Lamb Meatballs

Prep Time: 10 minutes| Cooking Time: 1 hour| Temperature: 250F|

Servings: 20

Ingredients:

- 1 lb. lamb shoulder, ground
- 3 garlic cloves, finely diced
- 3 tbsp. shallot, diced
- 1 tbsp. salt
- 1 egg
- 1/2 tbsp. pepper
- 1/2 tbsp. cumin
- 1/2 tbsp. smoked paprika
- 1/4 tbsp. red pepper flakes
- 1/4 tbsp. cinnamon
- 1/4 cup panko breadcrumbs

Directions:

1. Preheat the Traeger to 250F.
2. Combine all the ingredients in a bowl and mix well.
3. Form golf ball-sized meatballs and place them on a baking sheet.
4. Place the baking sheet in the smoker and smoke until the internal temperature reaches 160F.
5. Remove the meatballs from the smoker and serve.

NUTRITION:

Calories: 93|Fat: 5.9g| Carb: 4.8g| Protein: 5g

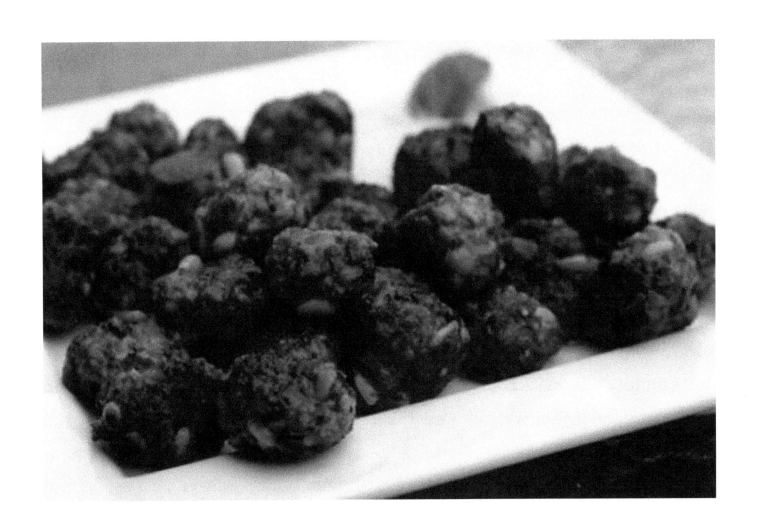

15. Traeger Crown Rack of Lamb

Prep Time: 30 minutes| Cooking Time: 30 minutes | Temperature: 450F| Servings: 6

Ingredients:

- 2 racks of lamb, frenched
- 1 tbsp garlic, crushed
- 1 tbsp rosemary
- 1/2 cup olive oil
- Kitchen twine

Directions:

1. Preheat the Traeger to 450F.
2. Rinse the lamb with cold water, then pat dry.
3. Lay the lamb flat on a chopping board and score a ¼ inch down between the bones. Repeat the process between the bones on each lamb rack. Set aside.
4. In a bowl, combine the garlic, rosemary, and oil. Brush the lamb with this mixture.
5. Bend the lamb rack into a semicircle, then place the frames together such that the bones will be up and will form a crown shape.
6. Wrap around 4 times, starting from the base moving upward. Tie tightly to keep the racks together.
7. Place the lambs on a baking sheet and set them in the Traeger. Cook on high heat for 10 minutes. Reduce the temperature to 300F and cook for 20 minutes more or until the internal temperature reaches 130F.
8. Remove the lamb rack from the Traeger and let rest

while wrapped in a foil for 15 minutes.

9. Serve.

NUTRITION:

Calories: 390 |Fat: 35g| Carb: 0g| Protein: 17g

Traeger Smoked Leg

Prep Time: 15 minutes | Cooking Time: 3 hours| Temperature: 250F|

Servings: 6

Ingredients:

- 1 leg of lamb, boneless
- 2 tbsp oil
- 4 garlic cloves, minced
- 2 tbsp oregano
- 1 tbsp thyme
- 2 tbsp salt
- 1 tbsp black pepper, freshly ground

Directions:

1. In a bowl, mix oil, garlic, and all the spices. Rub the mixture all over the lamb, then cover with a plastic wrap.
2. Place the lamb in a fridge and marinate for 1 hour.
3. Transfer the lamb on a smoker rack and set the Traeger to smoke at 250F.
4. Smoke the meat for 4 hours or until the internal temperature reaches 145F.
5. Remove from the Traeger and serve.

NUTRITION:

Calories: 356|Fat: 16g| Carb: 3g| Protein: 49g

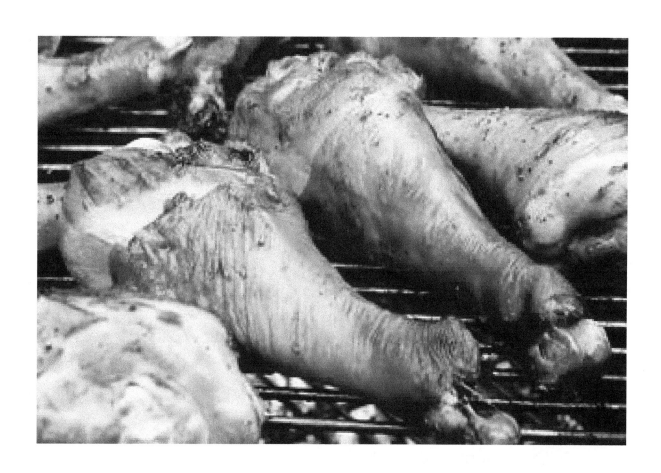

16. Traeger Grilled Aussie Leg of Lamb

Prep Time: 30 minutes | Cooking Time: 2 hours | Temperature: 350F|
Servings: 8

Ingredients:

- 5 lb. Aussie Boneless Leg of lamb

Smoked Paprika Rub

- 1 tbsp raw sugar
- 1 tbsp salt
- 1 tbsp black pepper
- 1 tbsp smoked paprika
- 1 tbsp garlic powder

- 1 tbsp rosemary
- 1 tbsp onion powder
- 1 tbsp cumin
- 1/2 tbsp cayenne pepper

Roasted Carrots

- 1 bunch rainbow carrots
- Olive oil as needed
- Salt and pepper to taste

Directions:

1. Preheat the Traeger to 350F.
2. Combine the paprika rub ingredients and rub the meat with this mixture.
3. Place the lamb on the preheated Traeger over indirect heat and smoke for 2 hours.
4. Meanwhile, toss the carrots in oil, salt, and pepper.
5. Add the carrots to the grill after 1 ½ hour or until the internal temperature has reached 90F.
6. Cook until the meat's internal temperature reaches 135F.
7. Remove the lamb from the Traeger and cover it with the foil for 30 minutes.
8. Serve.

NUTRITION:

Calories: 257|Fat: 8g| Carb: 6g| Protein: 37g

17. Lamb Chops

Prep Time: 15 minutes | Cooking Time: 30 minutes | Temperature: 240F| Servings: 4

Ingredients:

- 4 lamb shoulder chops
- 4 cup buttermilk
- 1 cup of cold water
- ¼ cup kosher salt
- 2 tbsp. olive oil
- 1 tbsp. Texas-style rub

Directions:

1. In a bowl, add the buttermilk, water, and salt and mix well.
2. Add the chops and coat with the mixture.
3. Refrigerate for at least 4 hours.
4. Remove the chops from the bowl and rinse under cold running water.
5. Coat the chops with olive oil and then sprinkle with rub evenly.
6. Preheat the Traeger to 240F with a closed lid for 15 minutes.
7. Arrange chops onto the grill and cook for 25 to 30 minutes or until desired doneness.
8. Meanwhile, preheat the broiler of the oven. Grease a broiler pan.
9. Remove the chops from the grill and place them onto the prepared broiler pan.
10. Transfer the broiler pan into the oven and broil for about 3 to 5 minutes or until browned.
11. Remove and serve.

NUTRITION:

Calories: 414 |Fat: 22.7g| Carb: 11.7g| Protein: 5.6g

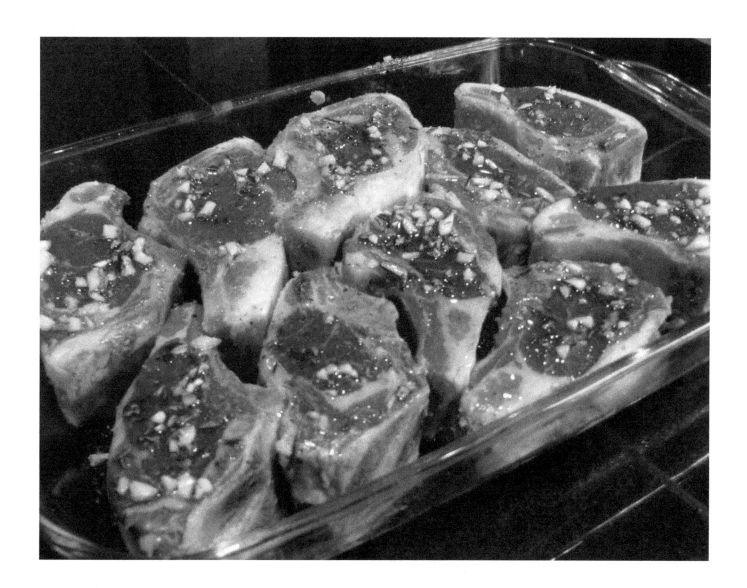

Lamb Chops

Prep Time: 10 minutes | Cooking Time: 12 minutes | Temperature: 450F| Servings: 6

Ingredients:

- o 6 (6-oz.) lamb chops
- o 3 tbsp. olive oil
- o Salt and ground black pepper, to taste

Directions:

1. Set the temperature of the Traeger to 450F and preheat with a closed lid for 15 minutes.
2. Coat the lamb chops with oil and season with salt and black pepper.
3. Arrange chops onto the grill and cook for 4 to 6 minutes per side.
4. Remove and serve.

NUTRITION:

Calories: 376|Fat: 19.5g| Carb: 0g| Protein: 47.8g

18. Lamb Chops

Prep Time: 15 minutes | Cooking Time: 17 minutes | Temperature: 500F| Servings: 4

Ingredients:

- ½ cup extra-virgin olive oil, divided
- ¼ cup onion, chopped roughly
- 2 garlic cloves, chopped roughly
- 2 tbsp. balsamic vinegar
- 2 tbsp. soy sauce
- 1 tsp. Worcestershire sauce
- 1 tbsp. fresh rosemary, chopped
- 2 tsp. Dijon mustard
- Ground black pepper, to taste
- 4 (5-oz.) lamb chops
- Salt, to taste

Directions:

1. Heat 1 tbsp. olive oil in a pan. Add onion and garlic and cook for 5 minutes.
2. Remove from the heat and transfer into a blender.
3. In the blender, add the vinegar, soy sauce, Worcestershire sauce, rosemary, mustard, and black pepper and pulse until well combined. Keep the motor running and slowly add the remaining oil and pulse until smooth.
4. Transfer the sauce into a bowl and set aside.
5. Preheat the grill to 500F with the lid closed for 15 minutes.
6. Coat the lamb chops with remaining oil and season with salt and black pepper.

7. Arrange the chops onto the grill and cook for 4 to 6 minutes per side.

8. Remove the chops from the grill and serve with the sauce.

NUTRITION:

Calories: 496|Fat: 35.8g| Carb: 2.8g| Protein:40.6g

19. Spicy Rack of Lamb

Prep Time: 15 minutes | Cooking Time: 3 hours | Temperature: 225F|
Servings: 6

Ingredients:

- 2 tbsp. paprika
- ½ tbsp. coriander seeds
- 1 tsp. cumin seeds
- 1 tsp. ground allspice
- 1 tsp. lemon peel powder
- Salt and ground black pepper, to taste
- 2 (1½-lb.) rack of lamb ribs, trimmed

Directions:

1. Set the temperature of Traeger to 225F and preheat with a closed lid for 15 minutes.
2. In a coffee grinder, add all ingredients except rib racks and grind them into a powder.
3. Coat the rib racks with a spice mixture.
4. Arrange the rib racks onto the grill and cook for 3 hours.
5. Remove the rib racks from the grill and place them onto a cutting board. Rest for 15 minutes.
6. Slice and serve.

NUTRITION:

Calories: 545|Fat: 29.7g| Carb: 1.7g| Protein: 64.4g

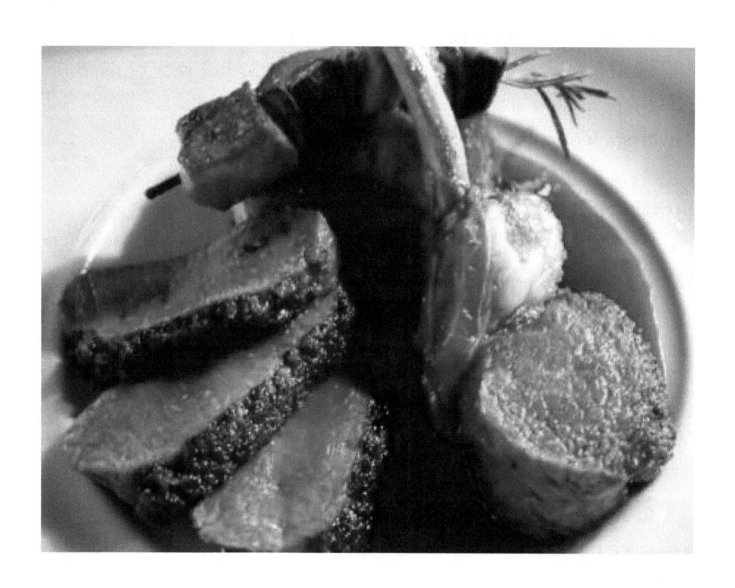

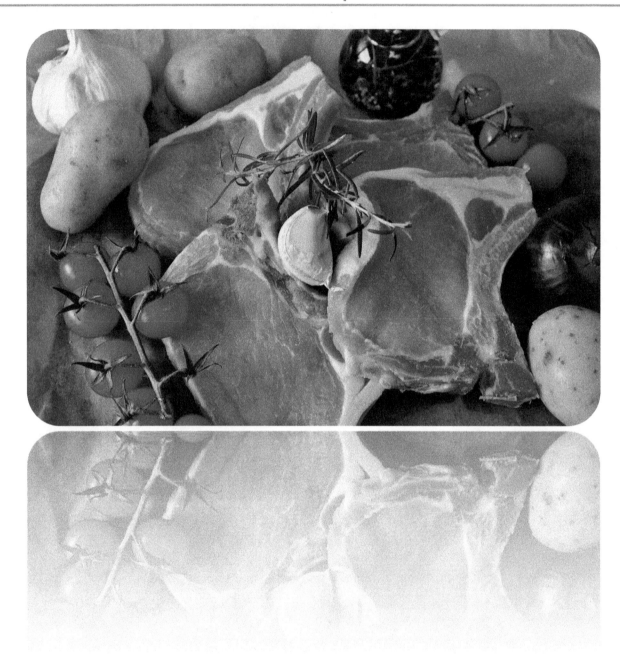

20. Pork Back Ribs

Prep Time: 15 minutes | Cooking Time: 5 hours | Temperature: 200F |
Servings: 16

Ingredients:

- ¼ cup yellow honey mustard
- ¼ cup brown sugar
- 1/3 cup paprika
- ¼ cup garlic powder
- ¼ cup onion powder
- 2 tbsp. chipotle chili pepper flakes
- 1 tbsp. ground cumin
- Salt and ground black pepper, to taste
- 2 tbsp. dried parsley flakes
- 8 lb. pork baby back ribs, silver skin removed

Directions:

1. In a bowl, add all ingredients except for ribs and mix well.
2. Rub the pork ribs with spice mixture.
3. Set the temperature of Traeger to 200F and preheat with a closed lid for 15 minutes.
4. Arrange the ribs onto the grill and cook for 2 hours.
5. Remove the ribs from the grill and wrap in heavy-duty foil.
6. Cook for 2 hours.
7. Remove the foil and cook for 1 hour more.
8. Remove from the grill and rest for 15 minutes.
9. Slice and serve.

NUTRITION:

Calories: 659 |Fat: 40.7g| Carb: 7.8g| Protein: 61.1g

21. BBQ Party Pork Ribs

Prep Time: 20 minutes| Cooking Time: 1 hour 55 minutes |
Temperature: 225F | Servings: 6

Ingredients:

- 2 bone-in racks of pork ribs, silver skin removed
- 6 oz. BBQ rub
- 8 oz. apple juice
- ½ cup BBQ sauce

Directions:

1. Coat each rack of ribs with BBQ rub generously.
2. Arrange the racks onto a platter and set aside for 30 minutes.
3. Set the temperature of Traeger to 225F and preheat with a closed lid for 15 minutes.
4. Arrange the racks onto the grill, bone side down, and cook for 1 hour.
5. Place apple juice in a spray bottle and spray the racks with vinegar mixture evenly.
6. Cook for 3 ½ hours, spraying with vinegar mixture after every 45 minutes.
7. Now, coat the racks with a thin layer of BBQ sauce evenly and cook for 10 minutes more.
8. Remove the racks from the grill and rest for 15 minutes.
9. Slice and serve.

NUTRITION:

Calories: 801|Fat: 40.6g| Carb: 44.9g| Protein: 60.4g

22. Summertime Pork Chops

Prep Time: 15 minutes | Cooking Time: 1 hour 35 minutes|
Temperature: 250F | Servings: 4

Ingredients:

For Brine:

- o 8 cups apple juice
- o 1 cup light brown sugar
- o ½ cup kosher salt
- o ½ cup BBQ rub

For Pork Chops:

- o 4 thick-cut pork loin chops
- o 2 tbsp. BBQ rub
- o 1 tbsp. Montreal steak seasoning

Directions:

1. For the brine: in a pan, add 4 cups of apple juice and cook until heated completely.

2. Add sugar, salt, and dry rub and cook until dissolved, stirring continuously.

3. Remove the pan from the heat and stir in the remaining apple juice. Set aside to cool completely.

4. In a large zip lock bag, add brine mixture and chops.

5. Seal the bag and refrigerate for about 2 hours.

6. Set the temperature of Traeger to 250F and preheat with a closed lid for 15 minutes.

7. Remove the chops from brine and set aside for 15 minutes.

8. Now, season the chops with BBQ rub and steak seasoning evenly.

9. Place the chops onto the grill and cook for 1 ½ hour.

10. Remove the chops from the grill and set aside for

about 5 minutes before 11. Serve.
serving.

NUTRITION:

Calories: 609|Fat: 12.6g| Carb: 92.6g| Protein: 29.5g

23. Pork Tenderloin

Prep Time: 10 minutes| Cooking Time: 3 hours | Temperature: 225F|
Servings: 6

Ingredients:

- ½ cup apple cider
- 3 tbsp. honey
- 2 (1¼-1½-lb.) pork tenderloins, silver skin removed
- 3 tbsp. sweet rub

Directions:

1. In a bowl, mix together apple cider and honey.
2. Coat the outside of tenderloins with honey mixture and season with the rub.
3. With a plastic wrap, cover each tenderloin and refrigerate for about 3 hours.
4. Set the temperature of Traeger to 225F and preheat with a closed lid for 15 minutes.
5. Arrange the tenderloins onto the grill and cook for 2 ½ to 3 hours.
6. Remove the pork tenderloins from the grill and rest for 10 minutes.
7. Slice and serve.

NUTRITION:

Calories: 498|Fat: 18.4g| Carb: 11.1g| Protein: 67.8g

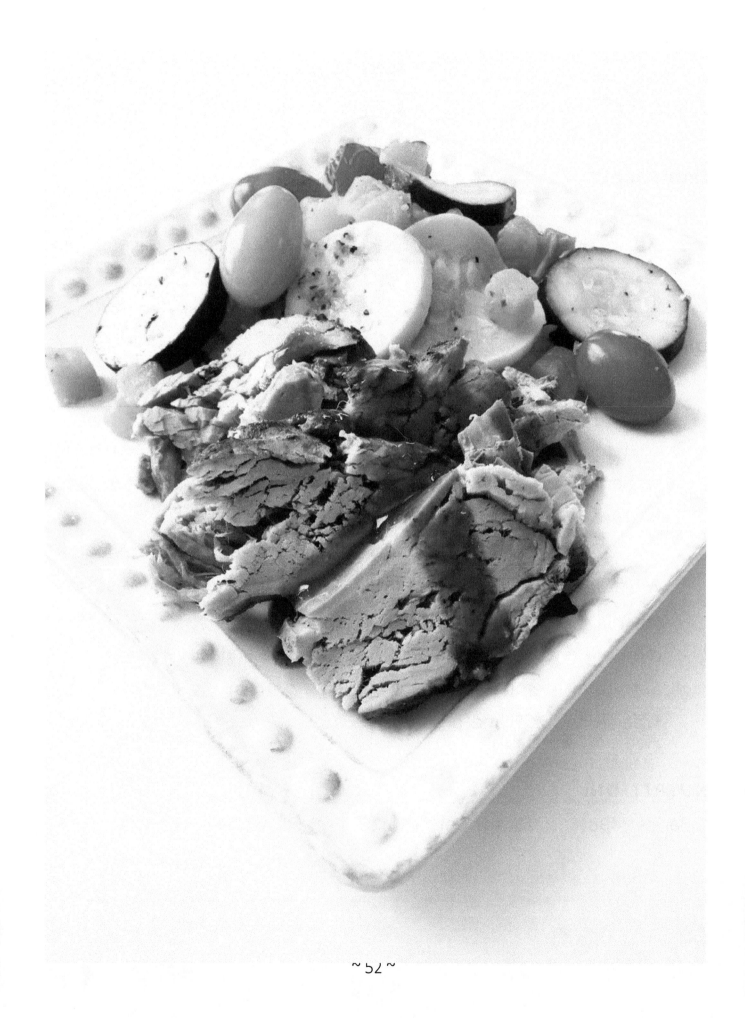

24. Pork Loin

Prep Time: 15 minutes | Cooking Time: 1 hour 40 minutes | Temperature: 350F| Servings: 8

Ingredients:

- 1 (12-oz.) bottle German lager
- 1/3 cup honey
- 2 tbsp. Dijon mustard
- 1 tsp. dried thyme
- 1 tsp. caraway seeds
- 1 (3-lb.) pork loin, silver skin removed
- 1 large Vidalia onion, chopped
- 3 garlic cloves, minced
- 3 tbsp. dry seasoned pork rub

Directions:

1. In a bowl, add the lager, honey, mustard, thyme, and caraway seeds and mix well.
2. In a Ziploc bag, place pork loin, onion, garlic, and honey mixture.
3. Seal the bag and shake to coat well. Refrigerate to marinate overnight.
4. Set the temperature of Traeger to 350F and preheat with a closed lid for 15 minutes.
5. Remove the pork loin, onions, and garlic from the bag and place onto a plate.
6. Rub the pork loin with pork rub evenly.
7. Place the seasoned pork, onions, and garlic into a large roasting pan.
8. Arrange the pork tenderloin, fat side pointing up.
9. Place the marinade into a pan over medium heat and bring to a boil.

10. Cook for 3 to 5 minutes or until the liquid reduces by half.

11. Remove from the heat and set aside.

12. Place the roasting pan onto the grill and cook for 1 hour.

13. Carefully pour the reduced marinade on top of the pork loin evenly.

14. Cook for 30 to 60 minutes more, basting the meat with marinade occasionally.

15. Remove from the grill and cool for 10 minutes.

16. Slice and serve.

NUTRITION:

Calories: 492|Fat: 23.9g| Carb: 16.3g| Protein: 47.2g

25. Pork Butt Roast

Prep Time: 10 minutes| Cooking Time: 14 hours | Temperature: 225F|

Servings: 14

Ingredients:

- ¼ cup brown sugar
- 2 tbsp. New Mexico chile powder
- 2 tbsp. garlic powder
- Salt, to taste
- 1 (7-lb.) fresh pork butt roast

Directions:

1. Set the temperature to Traeger to 225F and preheat with a closed lid for 15 minutes.
2. In a bowl, place all ingredients except for pork roast and mix well.
3. Rub the pork roast with spice mixture.
4. Arrange a roasting rack in a drip pan.
5. Place the pork roast onto the rack in a drip pan.
6. Place the drip pan onto the grill and cook for 8 to 14 hours or until the desired doneness.
7. Remove from grill and cool.
8. Slice and serve.

NUTRITION:

Calories: 439 |Fat: 28.3g| Carb: 4g| Protein: 40g

26. Fajita Favorite Pork Shoulder

Prep Time: 15 minutes| Cooking Time: 10 hours| Temperature: 160F & 250F | Servings: 20

Ingredients:

For Brine:

- o 4 cup hot water
- o 1 cup kosher salt
- o ¼ cup brown sugar
- o 2 tbsp. black peppercorn
- o 12 cups cold water
- o 8 cups apple cider
- o ¼ cup apple cider vinegar
- o ¼ cup Worcestershire sauce

For Pork:

- o 8½ pounds pork shoulder roast, trimmed
- o ¼-½ cup pork rub

Directions:

1. For the brine: in a container, add hot water, salt, brown sugar, and peppercorn and mix until dissolved.
2. Add the cold water, apple cider, vinegar, and Worcestershire sauce and mix until well combined.
3. Score the pork on both sides with a knife, then place it in the brine.
4. Cover the container and refrigerate for 24 hours.
5. Remove the pork from the container and discard the brine.
6. Rinse the pork shoulder under running cold water.
7. Pat dry the pork shoulder completely.
8. Place the pork shoulder onto a baking sheet and refrigerate for 2 hours or up to overnight.
9. Set the temperature of Traeger to 160F and preheat

with a closed lid for 15 minutes.

10. Place the pork shoulder onto the grill and cook for 4 hours.

11. Now, set the temperature of the gill to 250F and cook for 4 to 6 hours.

12. Remove the pork shoulder from the grill and place onto a baking sheet for about 40 to 60 minutes.

13. Shred the meat and serve.

NUTRITION:

Calories: 626|Fat: 41.4g| Carb: 15g| Protein: 45g

27. Pork Belly

Prep Time: 10 minutes | Cooking Time: 8 hours | Temperature: 225F|
Servings: 12

Ingredients:

o 1 (5-lb.) pork belly, skin removed

o Kosher salt and coarsely ground black pepper, to taste

Directions:

1. Set the temperature of Traeger to 225F and preheat with a closed lid for 15 minutes.
2. Rub the pork belly with salt and black pepper.
3. Arrange the pork belly onto the grill and cook for 6 to 8 hours.
4. Remove the pork belly from the grill and cool for 15 minutes.
5. Serve.

NUTRITION:

Calories: 534|Fat: 46.7g| Carb: 0g| Protein: 28.9g

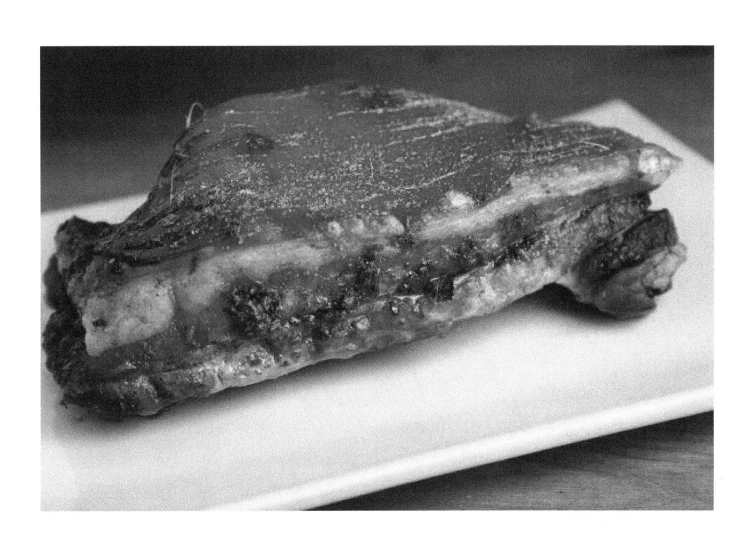

28. Christmas Ham

Prep Time: 15 minutes | Cooking Time: 1 hour 20 minutes |
Temperature: 325F| Servings: 16

Ingredients:

- 1 cup honey
- ¼ cup dark corn syrup
- 1 (7-lb.) ready-to-eat ham
- ¼ cup whole cloves
- ½ cup butter softened

Directions:

1. Set the temperature of Traeger to 325F and preheat with a closed lid for 15 minutes.
2. In a pan, add honey and corn syrup and cook until heated slightly, stirring continuously.
3. Remove the pan of glaze from heat and set aside.
4. Score the ham in a cross pattern with a knife.
5. Insert whole cloves at the crossings.
6. Coat the ham with butter evenly.
7. Arrange ham in a foil-lined roasting pan and top with ¾ of glaze evenly.
8. Place the pan onto the grill and cook for 1 ¼ hour, coating with remaining glaze after every 10 to 15 minutes.
9. Remove the ham from the grill and cool for 25 minutes.
10.   Slice and serve.

NUTRITION:

Calories: 457|Fat: 23.1g| Carb: 29.7g| Protein: 33.2g

29. Grilled Pork Chops

Prep Time: 15 minutes | Cooking Time: 20 minutes | Temperature: 450F| Servings: 6

Ingredients:

- 6 thick-cut pork chops
- BBQ rub as needed

Directions:

1. Preheat the Traeger to 450F.
2. Season the pork chops with the BBQ rub.
3. Place the chops on the Traeger and cook for 6 minutes on each side or until the internal temperature reaches 145F.
4. Remove the chops from the Traeger and cool for 5 minutes.
5. Serve.

NUTRITION:

Calories: 398|Fat: 19g| Carb: 8g| Protein: 46g

30. Traeger Bacon

Prep Time: 5 minutes | Cooking Time: 25 minutes | Temperature: 375F| Servings: 6

Ingredients:

- o 1 lb. bacon

Directions:

1. Preheat the Traeger to 375F.
2. Line a baking sheet with parchment paper, then arrange the thick-cut bacon on it in a single layer.
3. Bake the bacon in the Traeger for 20 minutes. Flip the bacon and cook for 20 minutes or until the bacon is no longer floppy.
4. Serve.

NUTRITION:

Calories: 315|Fat: 10g| Carb: 0g| Protein: 9g

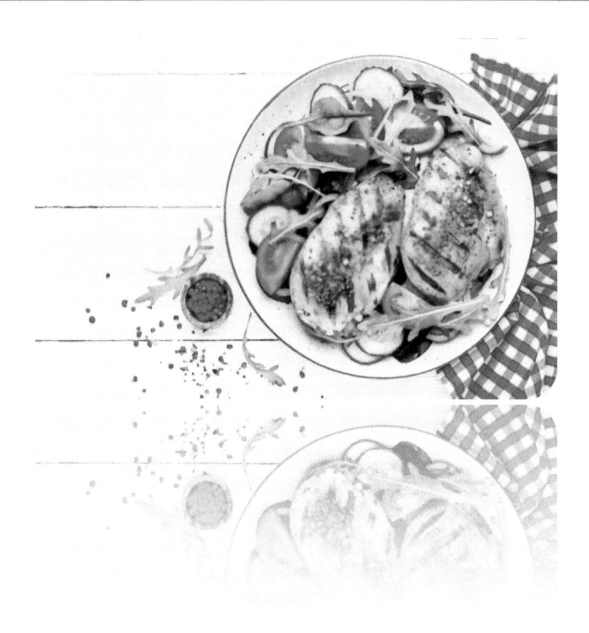

31. Traeger Grilled Chicken

Prep Time: 10 minutes | Cooking Time: 1 hour 10 minutes|
Temperature: 450F| Servings: 6

Ingredients:

- 5 lb. whole chicken
- 1/2 cup oil
- Traeger chicken rub

Directions:

1. Preheat the Traeger to 450F for 15 minutes with lid closed.
2. Use bakers' twine to tie the chicken legs together, then rub it with oil. Coat the chicken with the rub and place it on the grill.
3. Grill for 70 minutes with the lid closed or until it reaches an internal temperature of 165F. Remove the chicken from the Traeger and rest for 15 minutes.
4. Cut and serve.

NUTRITION:

Calories: 935|Fat: 53g| Carb: 0g| Protein: 107g

32. Traeger Chicken Breast

Prep Time: 10 minutes | Cooking Time: 15 minutes | Temperature: 375F| Servings: 6

Ingredients:

- o 3 chicken breasts
- o 1 tbsp avocado oil
- o 1/4 tbsp garlic powder
- o 1/4 tbsp onion powder
- o 3/4 tbsp salt
- o 1/4 tbsp pepper

Directions:

1. Preheat the Traeger to 375F.
2. Cut the chicken breast into halves lengthwise, then coat with avocado oil.
3. Season with garlic powder, onion powder, salt, and pepper.
4. Place the chicken on the grill and cook for 7 minutes on each side or until the internal temperature reaches 165F.
5. Serve.

NUTRITION:

Calories: 120|Fat: 4g| Carb: 0g| Protein: 19g

33. Smoked Spatchcock Turkey

Prep Time: 30 minutes | Cooking Time: 1 hour 15 minutes | Temperature: 400F & 300F| Servings: 8

Ingredients:

- 1 turkey
- 1/2 cup melted butter
- 1/4 cup Traeger chicken rub
- 1 tbsp onion powder
- 1 tbsp garlic powder
- 1 tbsp rubbed sage

Directions:

1. Preheat the Traeger to 400F.
2. Place the turkey on a chopping board with the breast side down and the legs pointing towards you.
3. Cut either side of the turkey backbone to remove the spine. Flip the turkey and place it on a pan.
4. Season both sides with the seasonings and place it on the grill skin side up on the grill.
5. Cook for 30 minutes, reduce temperature to 300F, and cook for 45 minutes more or until the internal temperature reaches 165F.
6. Remove from the grill and rest for 15 minutes.
7. Slice and serve.

NUTRITION:

Calories: 156|Fat: 16g| Carb: 1g| Protein: 22g

34. Smoked Cornish Hens

Prep Time: 10 minutes | Cooking Time: 1 hour | Temperature: 275F | Servings: 6

Ingredients:

- 6 Cornish hens
- 3 tbsp oil
- 6 tbsp rub (your choice)

Directions:

1. Preheat the Traeger to 275F.
2. Meanwhile, rub the hens with oil and then with your favorite rub.
3. Place the hens on the grill with the breast side down. Smoke for 30 minutes.
4. Flip the hens and increase the Traeger temperature to 400F. Cook until the internal temperature reaches 165F.
5. Remove the hens from the grill and rest for 10 minutes.
6. Serve.

NUTRITION:

Calories: 696|Fat: 50g| Carb:1g | Protein:57g

35. Smoked and Fried Chicken Wings

Prep Time: 10 minutes | Cooking Time: 2 hours | Temperature: 180F|

Servings: 4

Ingredients:

- 3 lb. chicken wings
- 1 tbsp adobo seasoning
- Your favorite sauce

Directions:

1. Preheat the Traeger to 180F.
2. Generously coat the wings with adobo seasoning and then place them on the grill.
3. Smoke them for 2 hours, turning them at least once during smoking.
4. Remove the wings from the smoker and heat oil to 375F.
5. Drop the wings in the hot oil and fry for 5 minutes or until the skin is crispy.
6. Remove the wings from the oil and drain.
7. Toss in your favorite sauce and serve.

NUTRITION:

Calories: 755|Fat: 55g| Carb: 24g| Protein: 39g

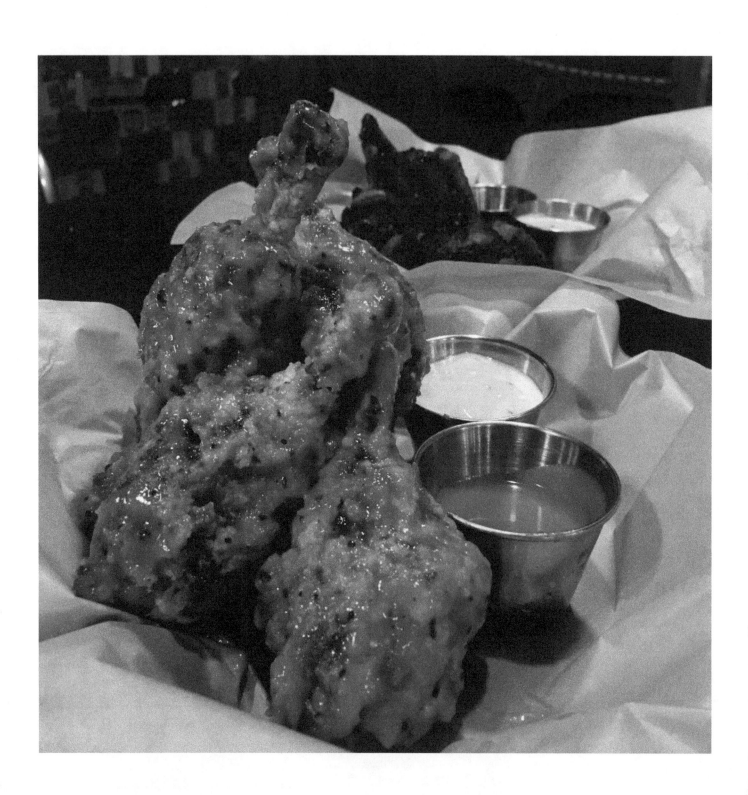

36. Grilled Buffalo Chicken Legs

Prep Time: 30 minutes | Cooking Time: 1 hour 15 minutes | Temperature: 325F| Servings: 8

Ingredients:

- 12 chicken legs
- 1/2 tbsp salt
- 1 tbsp buffalo seasoning
- 1 cup Buffalo sauce

Directions:

1. Preheat the Traeger to 325F.
2. Toss the chicken legs in salt and seasoning, then place them on the preheated grill.
3. Grill for 40 minutes, turning twice.
4. Increase the heat to 375F and cook for 10 minutes more. Brush the chicken legs and brush with buffalo sauce.
5. Cook for 10 minutes more, or the internal temperature reaches 165F.
6. Remove from the Traeger and brush with more buffalo sauce.
7. Serve.

NUTRITION:

Calories: 956 |Fat: 47g| Carb: 1g| Protein: 124g

37. Traeger Chili Lime Chicken

Prep Time: 2 minutes | Cooking Time: 15 minutes | Temperature: 400F|

Servings: 1

Ingredients:

o 1 chicken breast

o 1 tbsp oil

o 1 tbsp Chile Lime Seasoning

Directions:

1. Preheat the Traeger to 400F.
2. Brush the chicken breast with oil, then sprinkle the chili-lime seasoning and salt.
3. Place the chicken breast on the grill and cook for 7 minutes on each side or until the internal temperature reaches 165F.
4. Serve.

NUTRITION:

Calories: 131|Fat: 5g| Carb: 4g| Protein: 19g

38. Grilled Buffalo Chicken

Prep Time: 5 minutes| Cooking Time: 20 minutes | Temperature: 400F|

Servings: 6

Ingredients:

- o 5 chicken breasts, boneless and skinless
- o 2 tbsp homemade BBQ rub
- o 1 cup homemade Cholula Buffalo sauce

Directions:

1. Preheat the Traeger to 400F.
2. Slice the chicken breast lengthwise into strips. Season the slices with BBQ rub.
3. Place the chicken slices on the grill and paint both sides with buffalo sauce.
4. Cook for 4 minutes with the lid closed. Flip the breasts, paint again with sauce and cook until the internal temperature reaches 165F.
5. Remove the chicken from the Traeger and serve.

NUTRITION:

Calories: 176|Fat: 4g| Carb: 1g| Protein: 32g

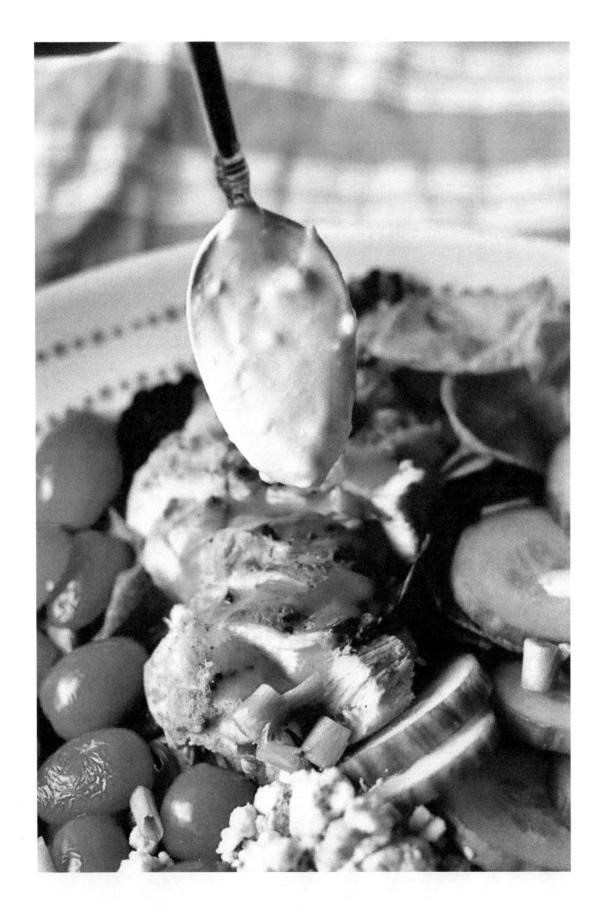

39. Sheet Pan Chicken Fajitas

Prep Time: 10 minutes | Cooking Time: 10 minutes | Temperature: 450F | Servings: 10

Ingredients:

- 2 lb. chicken breast
- 1 onion, sliced
- 1 red bell pepper, seeded and sliced
- 1 orange-red bell pepper, seeded and sliced
- 1 tbsp salt
- 1/2 tbsp onion powder
- 1/2 tbsp granulated garlic
- 2 tbsp Chile Margarita Seasoning
- 2 tbsp oil

Directions:

1. Preheat the Traeger to 450F and line a baking sheet with parchment paper.
2. In a bowl, combine seasonings and oil, then toss with the peppers and chicken.
3. Place the baking sheet in the Traeger and let heat for 10 minutes with the lid closed.
4. Open the lid and place the veggies and the chicken in a single layer.
5. Close the lid and cook for 10 minutes or until the chicken is no longer pink.
6. Serve.

NUTRITION:

Calories: 211|Fat: 6g| Carb: 5g| Protein: 29g

40. Asian Miso Chicken Wings

Prep Time: 15 minutes | Cooking Time: 25 minutes | Temperature: 375F| Servings: 6

Ingredients:

- 2 lb. chicken wings
- 3/4 cup soy
- 1/2 cup pineapple juice
- 1 tbsp sriracha
- 1/8 cup miso
- 1/8 cup gochujang
- 1/2 cup water
- 1/2 cup oil
- Togarashi

Directions:

1. Preheat the Traeger to 375F.
2. Combine all the ingredients except Togarashi in a zip lock bag. Toss until the chicken wings are coated. Refrigerate for 12 hours.
3. Place the wings on the grill grates and close the lid. Cook for 25 minutes or until the internal temperature reaches 165F.
4. Remove the wings from the Traeger and sprinkle Togarashi.
5. Serve.

NUTRITION:

Calories: 703|Fat: 56g| Carb: 23g| Protein: 27g

41. Special Occasion's Dinner Cornish Hen

Prep Time: 15 minutes | Cooking Time: 1 hour| Temperature: 375F|
Servings: 4

Ingredients:

- 4 Cornish game hens
- 4 fresh rosemary sprigs
- 4 tbsp. butter, melted
- 4 tsp. chicken rub

Directions:

1. Set the temperature to Traeger Grill to 375F and preheat with a closed lid for 15 minutes.
2. Pat dry the hens with paper towels.
3. Tuck the wings behind the backs, and with kitchen strings, tie the legs together.
4. Coat the outside of each hen with melted butter and sprinkle with rub evenly.
5. Stuff the cavity of each hen with a rosemary sprig.
6. Place the hens onto the grill and cook for 50 to 60 minutes.
7. Remove the hens from the grill and place onto a platter for about 10 minutes.
8. Cut and serve.

NUTRITION:

Calories: 430|Fat: 33g| Carb: 2.1g| Protein: 25.4g

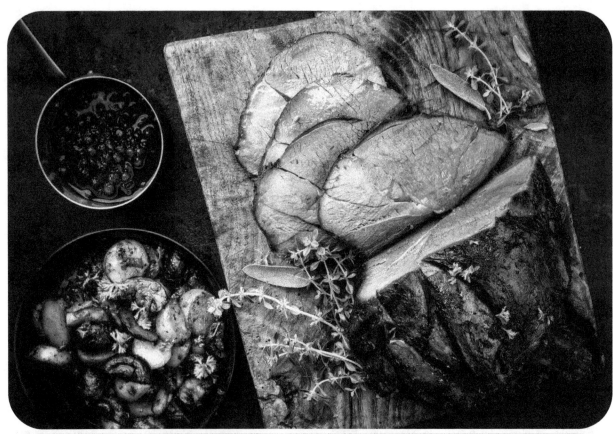

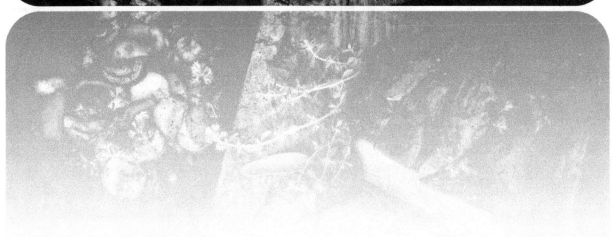

42. Wild Elk Tenderloin Kabobs

Prep Time: 15 minutes | Cooking Time: 15 minutes | Temperature: 500F| Servings: 8

Ingredients:

- 3 lb. elk tenderloin, cut into 2-inch chunks
- 3 tbsp balsamic vinegar
- 3 tbsp olive oil
- 3 yellow squash, whole
- 3 zucchinis, whole
- 12 sweet peppers, small
- 12 cherry tomatoes
- 2 tbsp Traeger prime rib rub

Directions:

1. Drizzle elk tenderloin chunks with vinegar and oil, and then let sit in a bowl.
2. Meanwhile, chop squash and zucchini into ¾-inch thick coins.
3. Now cut ends off from the peppers and remove seeds.
4. Place peppers, tomatoes, zucchini, and squash coins in the bowl with tenderloin, then toss them. Add more vinegar and oil until everything is lightly coated.
5. Now generously add rib rub and continue tossing.
6. Stack meat and vegetables, alternating them onto the skewer.
7. In the meantime, preheat the Traeger to 500F with the lid closed for 15 minutes.
8. Place the kabobs on the grate directly and grill for 15 minutes.
9. Serve.

NUTRITION:

Calories: 349|Fat: 9.7g| Carb: 20.7g| Protein: 46g

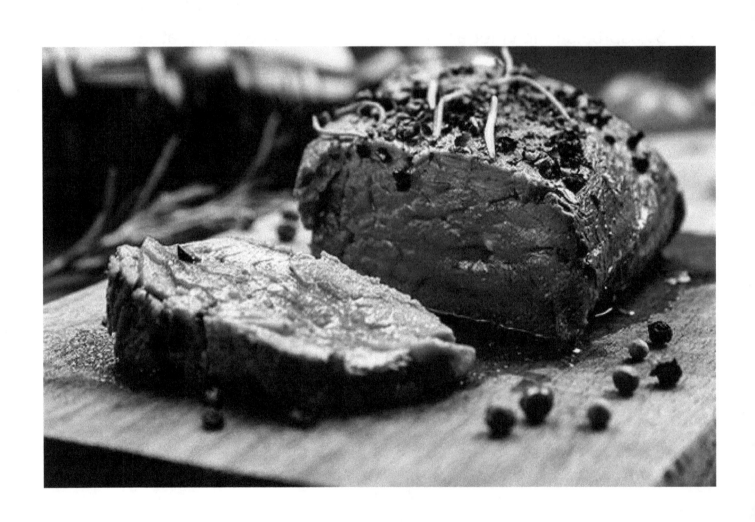

43. Smoked Venison Tenderloin

Prep Time: 5 minutes | Cooking Time: 2 hours| Temperature: 275F|
Servings: 4

Ingredients:

- 1 lb. venison tenderloin
- 1/4 cup lemon juice
- 1/4 cup olive oil
- 5 garlic cloves
- 1 tbsp salt
- 1 tbsp black pepper, ground + more for serving

Directions:

1. Place venison tenderloins in a bowl.
2. Process all the other ingredients in a blender until broken into small pieces and mixed well.
3. Pour and massage the marinade over the venison and refrigerate it for about 4 hours or overnight.
4. Now remove venison tenderloins from the marinade, rinse, pat dry, and cool at room temperature for 30 minutes.
5. Preheat the Traeger to 275F.
6. Place the venison on your Traeger and smoke for 2 hours or until nice and juicily. Make sure the internal temperature reaches 130F to 140F for rare and medium-rare, respectively.
7. Slice and top with more pepper.
8. Remove and rest for 10 minutes.
9. Serve.

NUTRITION:

Calories: 290|Fat: 15.5g| Carb: 2.6g| Protein: 34.5g

44. Grilled Quail, South Carolina Style

Prep Time: 20 minutes | Cooking Time: 20 minutes | Temperature: 400F| Servings: 4

Ingredients:

- o 4 tbsp butter
- o 1/2 grated onion
- o 3-4 tbsp vegetable oil
- o 1/2 cup yellow mustard
- o 1/2 cup sugar, brown
- o 1/2 cup cider vinegar
- o 1 tbsp dry mustard
- o 1 tbsp cayenne
- o Salt to taste
- o 8-16 quails

Directions:

1. Melt butter in a pan and sauté onions for 4 minutes.
2. Add all other ingredients except quails and simmer for 20 minutes. Simmer slowly.
3. Buzz in a blender to make a smooth sauce.
4. Flatten and remove quail's backbone by cutting along the side using kitchen shears. Place the quails on a cutting board with the breast side up, then press them to flatten.
5. Meanwhile, preheat the Traeger to 400F and place the quails with the breast side up.
6. Grill the quails with the lid closed for about 5 minutes. Rub the breast side using your sauce as it cooks.
7. Turn over the quails and grill for another 2 minutes with the lid open.

8. Turn over again and rub with sauce once more, cover your Traeger and cook for 2 to 4 minutes.

9. Remove quails from the Traeger and rub with sauce once more.

NUTRITION:

Calories: 673|Fat: 40g| Carb: 9g| Protein: 45g

45. Traeger Grilled Rabbit

Prep Time: 5 minutes| Cooking Time: 40 minutes| Temperature: 500F & 425F| Servings: 8

Ingredients:

- o 1 whole rabbit fryer
- o 1 cup spicy plum sauce

For grilling:

- o Assorted veggies

Directions:

1. Preheat the grill to 500F.
2. In the meantime, cut the rabbit rib cage pressing down flat.
3. Spread half of the sauce on the rabbit inside, then lay the rabbit on the grill with marinade side down.
4. Lower the heat to 425F. Cover and cook for 15 to 20 minutes.
5. Then coat the rabbit's top side with the remaining sauce and flip the rabbit, then coat with the sauce.
6. Add assorted veggies and cover the grill. Cook for 15 to 20 minutes more or until the internal temperature reads 160F and all juices run clear.
7. Remove and rest for 10 minutes.
8. Chop and serve.

NUTRITION:

Calories: 115|Fat: 4.6g| Carb: 1g| Protein: 16.5g

46. Smoked Doves

Prep Time: 30 minutes| Cooking Time: 2 hours| Temperature: 200F|
Servings: 10

Ingredients:

- 1/2 cup kosher salt
- 2 quarts water
- 16-20 doves
- 1 tbsp Instacure No 1

For guajillo sauce

- 5 unpeeled garlic cloves
- 1 quartered white onion, small and roughly chopped
- 2-5 hot chiles
- 8 guajillo peppers, dried and stems/seeds removed
- 2 tbsp tomato paste
- 1 tbsp Mexican oregano, dried
- 1/4 tbsp allspice
- 1/4 tbsp coriander, ground
- Salt to taste
- Lime juice to taste

Directions:

1. Dissolve salt in water and then submerge the doves in the water. Refrigerate for about 4 hours. Now remove from the fridge, rinse and pat them dry.
2. Preheat the Traeger to 200F.
3. Place the doves on the Traeger and smoke for 2 hours.
4. In the meantime, rehydrate chiles by pouring boiling water over them.
5. Char garlic and onions in a dry skillet, hot, until nice blackening. Now peel the garlic and place both onions and garlic in a blender.
6. Add chiles and remaining sauce ingredients into the blender. Process until

smooth while adjusting seasoning with lime juice and salt.

7. Remove the doves from the grill, half them using kitchen shears, and coat with the sauce.

8. Serve.

NUTRITION:

Calories: 610|Fat: 19.7g| Carb: 3.6g| Protein: 101.2g

47. Smoked Pheasant

Prep Time: 15 minutes | Cooking Time: 1 hour 45 minutes|
Temperature: 275F| Servings: 3

Ingredients:

- 3 whole pheasant
- 3 tbsp smoky rooster booster rub
- Traeger Saskatchewan rub as needed
- 1 quartered red bell pepper, whole, and core removed
- 1 white onion, whole and sliced into thin sections
- 4 tbsp olive oil
- Pepper to taste
- Salt to taste
- 1 whole box rice pilaf

Directions:

1. Preheat the Traeger to 275F while the lid closed for about 10 to 15 minutes.
2. Clean pheasant thighs and breasts, then rinse and place in a zip lock bag.
3. Add rooster booster rub and a generous amount of Traeger Saskatchewan rub. Shake well and set aside.
4. Brush pepper and onions lightly using oil, then splash with pepper and salt. Place them on a tin foil and to one side of the grill.
5. Smoke the veggies for about 1 hour, then place your pheasant on the grill.
6. Cook for 30 to 45 minutes.
7. Remove and serve with rice pilaf.

NUTRITION:

Calories: 926|Fat: 24.9g| Carb: 4.8g| Protein: 161g

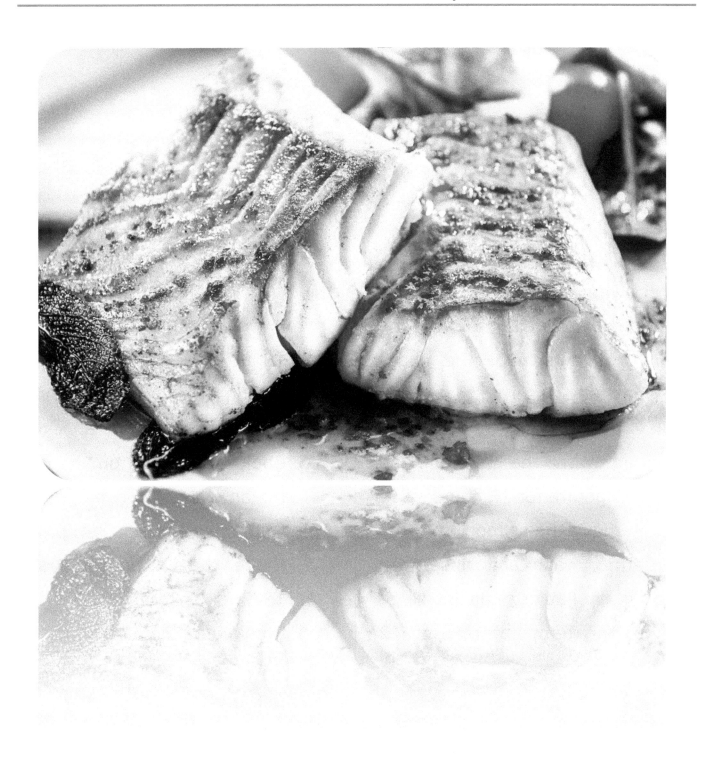

48. Wood Pellet Smoked Salmon

Prep Time: 10 minutes| Cooking Time: 4 hours | Temperature: 180F|
Servings: 8

Ingredients:

Brine

- o 4 cups of water
- o 1 cup brown sugar
- o 1/3 cup kosher salt

Salmon

- o 4 lb. salmon fillet, skin in
- o Maple syrup

Directions:

1. Combine all the brine ingredients until the sugar has fully dissolved.
2. Add the brine to a Ziplock bag with the salmon and refrigerate for 12 hours.
3. Remove the salmon from the brine, wash and rinse with water. Pat dry and let sit at room temperature for 2 hours.
4. Preheat the grill to smoke 180F. Place the salmon on a baking rack sprayed with cooking spray.
5. Cook the salmon on the grill for an hour. Then baste the salmon with maple syrup. Do the let the smoker get above 180F.
6. Smoke for 3 to 4 hours or until salmon flakes easily.
7. Serve.

NUTRITION:

Calories: 101|Fat: 2g | Carb: 16g| Protein: 4g

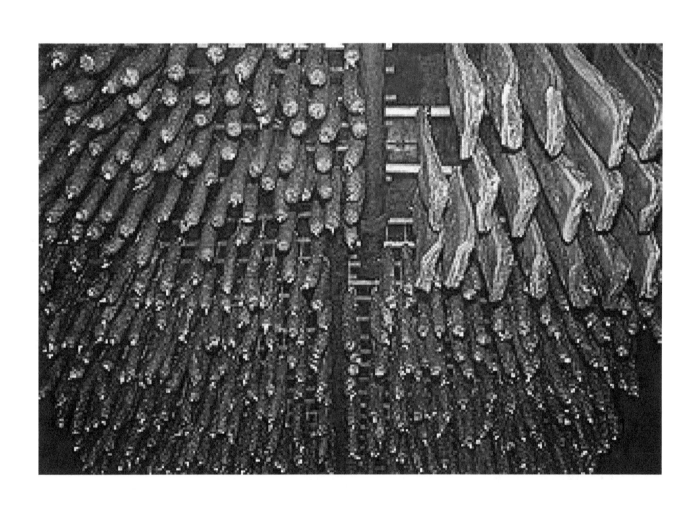

49. Teriyaki Smoked Shrimp

Prep Time: 10 minutes | Cooking Time: 10 minutes | Temperature: 450F| Servings: 6

Ingredients:

- 1 lb. tail-on shrimp, uncooked
- 1/2 tbsp onion powder
- 1/2 tbsp salt
- 1/2 tbsp Garlic powder
- 4 tbsp Teriyaki sauce
- 4 tbsp sriracha mayo
- 2 tbsp green onion, minced

Directions:

1. Peel the shrimps leaving the tails, then wash them, removing any vein left over. Drain and pat with a paper towel to drain.
2. Preheat the grill to 450F.
3. Season the shrimp with onion, salt, and garlic, then place it on the grill to cook for 5 minutes on each side.
4. Remove the shrimp from the grill and toss it with Teriyaki sauce.
5. Serve garnished with mayo and onions.

NUTRITION:

Calories: 87|Fat: 0g| Carb: 2g | Protein: 16g

50. Grilled Scallops

Prep Time: 5 minutes | Cooking Time: 15 minutes| Temperature: 400F| Servings: 4

Ingredients:

- 2 lb. sea scallops, dried with a paper towel
- 1/2 tbsp garlic salt
- 2 tbsp kosher salt
- 4 tbsp salted butter
- Squeeze lemon juice

Directions:

1. Preheat the grill to 400F with the cast pan inside.
2. Sprinkle with both salts, pepper on both sides of the scallops.
3. Place the butter on the cast iron, then add the scallops. Close the lid and cook for 8 minutes.
4. Flip the scallops and close the lid once more. Cook for 8 minutes more.
5. Remove the scallops from the rill and give a lemon squeeze. Serve.

NUTRITION:

Calories: 177|Fat: 7g| Carb: 6g | Protein: 23g

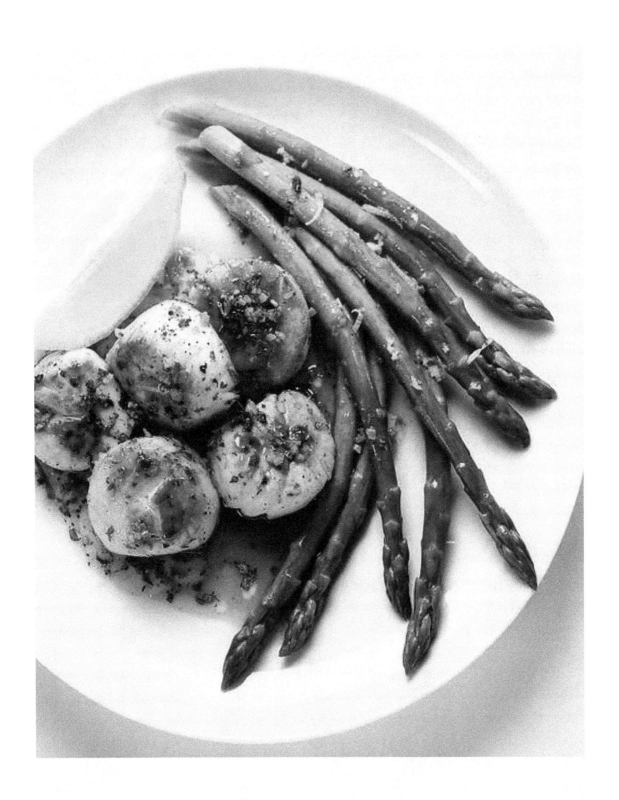

51. Grilled Shrimp Scampi

Prep Time: 5 minutes | Cooking Time: 10 minutes | Temperature: 400F|
Servings: 4

Ingredients:

- o 1 lb. raw shrimp, tail on
- o 1/2 cup salted butter, melted
- o 1/4 cup white wine, dry
- o 1/2 tbsp fresh garlic, chopped
- o 1 tbsp lemon juice
- o 1/2 tbsp garlic powder
- o 1/2 tbsp salt

Directions:

1. Preheat the grill to 400F with a cast iron inside.
2. In a bowl, mix butter, wine, garlic, and juice, then pour in the cast iron. Let the mixture mix for 4 minutes.
3. Sprinkle garlic and salt on the shrimp, then place it on the cast iron. Grill for 10 minutes with the lid closed.
4. Remove the shrimp from the grill and serve.

NUTRITION:

Calories: 298|Fat: 24g| Carb: 2g| Protein: 16g

52. Smoked Buffalo Shrimp

Prep Time: 10 minutes | Cooking Time: 5 minutes | Temperature: 450F|
Servings: 6

Ingredients:

- 1 lb. raw shrimps peeled and deveined
- 1/2 tbsp salt
- 1/4 tbsp garlic salt
- 1/4 tbsp garlic powder
- 1/4 tbsp onion powder
- 1/2 cup buffalo sauce

Directions:

1. Preheat the grill to 450F.
2. Coat the shrimp salt, garlic, and onion powders.
3. Place the shrimp on a grill and cook for 3 minutes on each side.
4. Remove from the grill and toss in buffalo sauce.
5. Serve.

NUTRITION:

Calories: 57|Fat: 1g| Carb: 1g| Protein: 10g

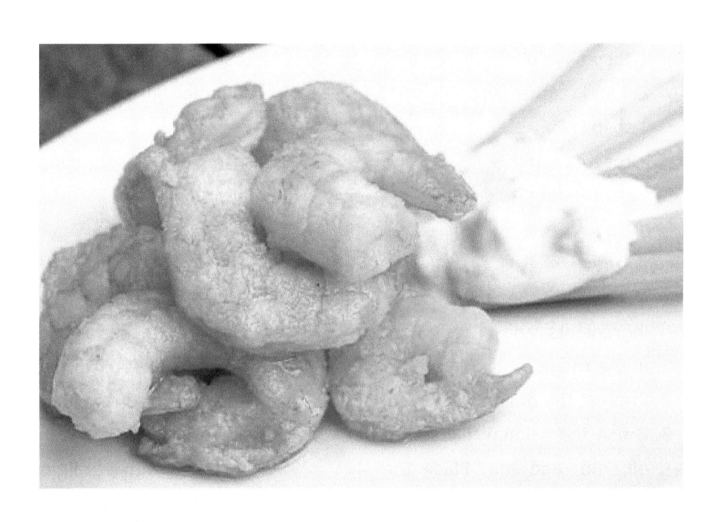

53. Grilled Salmon Sandwich

Prep Time: 10 minutes | Cooking Time: 15 minutes | Temperature: 450F| Servings: 4

Ingredients:

Salmon Sandwiches

- o 4 salmon fillets
- o 1 tbsp olive oil
- o Fin and feather rub
- o 1 tbsp salt
- o 4 toasted buns
- o Butter lettuce

Dill Aioli

- o 1/2 cup mayonnaise
- o 1/2 tbsp lemon zest
- o 2 tbsp lemon juice
- o 1/4 tbsp salt
- o 1/2 tbsp fresh dill, minced

Directions:

1. Mix all the dill aioli ingredients and place them in the fridge.
2. Preheat the grill to 450F.
3. Brush the salmon fillets with oil, rub, and salt. Place the fillets on the grill and cook until the internal temperature reaches 135F.
4. Remove the fillets from the grill and rest for 5 minutes.
5. Spread the aioli on the buns, then top with salmon, lettuce, and the top bun. Serve.

NUTRITION:

Calories: 852|Fat: 54g| Carb: 30g| Protein: 57g

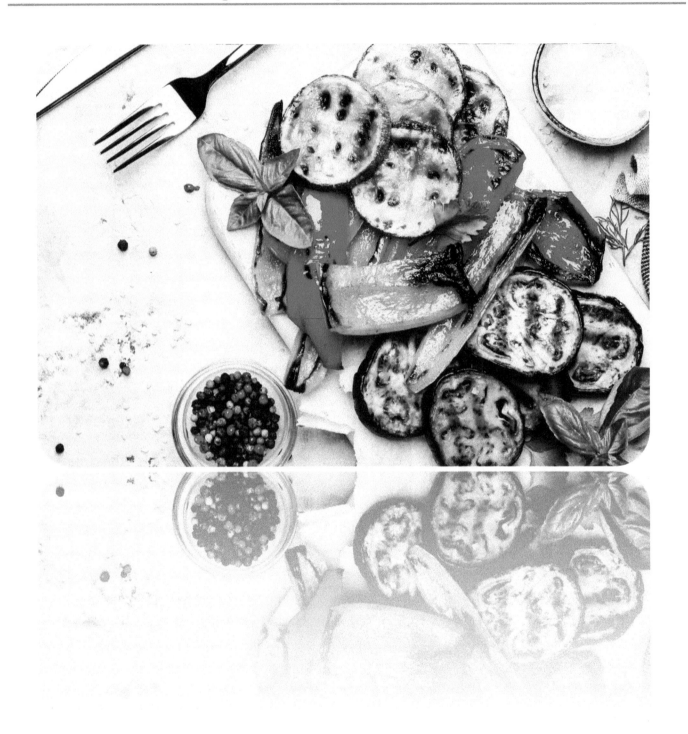

54. Smoked Mushrooms

Prep Time: 15 minutes | Cooking Time: 45 minutes | Temperature: 180F & 400F| Servings: 5

Ingredients:

- o 4 cups portobello, whole and cleaned
- o 1 tbsp oil
- o 1 tbsp onion powder
- o 1 tbsp granulated garlic
- o 1 tbsp salt
- o 1 tbsp pepper

Directions:

1. In a bowl, add all ingredients and mix well.
2. Set the grill to 180F and place the mushrooms directly on the grill.
3. Smoke the mushrooms for 30 minutes.
4. Increase the temperature to 400F and cook the mushrooms for 15 minutes more.
5. Serve.

NUTRITION:

Calories: 168|Fat: 3g| Carb: 10g| Protein: 4g

55. Grilled Zucchini Squash Spears

Prep Time: 5 minutes | Cooking Time: 10 minutes | Temperature: 350F|
Servings: 5

Ingredients:

- 4 zucchinis, cleaned and ends cut
- 2 tbsp olive oil
- 1 tbsp sherry vinegar
- 2 thyme, leaves pulled
- Salt and pepper to taste

Directions:

1. Cut zucchinis into halves, then cut each half thirds.
2. Add the rest of the ingredients in a zip lock bag with the zucchini pieces. Mix well.
3. Set the grill temperature to 350F with the lid closed for 15 minutes.
4. Remove the zucchini from the bag and place them on the grill grate with the cut side down.
5. Cook for 4 minutes per side or until zucchini are tender.
6. Remove from the grill and serve with thyme leaves.

NUTRITION:

Calories: 74|Fat: 5.4g| Carb: 6.1g| Protein: 2.6g

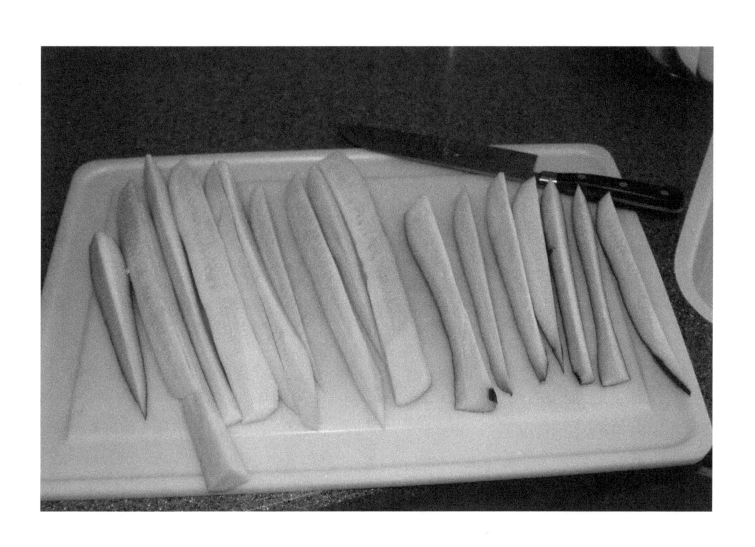

56. Grilled Asparagus and Honey Glazed Carrots

Prep Time: 15 minutes | Cooking Time: 35 minutes | Temperature: 165F| Servings: 5

Ingredients:

- 1 bunch asparagus, trimmed ends
- 1 lb. carrots, peeled
- 2 tbsp olive oil
- Sea salt to taste
- 2 tbsp honey
- Lemon zest

Directions:

1. Sprinkle the asparagus with oil and sea salt. Drizzle the carrots with honey and salt.
2. Set the grill temperature to 165F and preheat with lid closed for 15 minutes.
3. Place the carrots in the grill and cook for 15 minutes. Add asparagus and cook for 20 minutes more or until cooked through.
4. Top the carrots and asparagus with lemon zest. Enjoy.

NUTRITION:

Calories:168 |Fat: 3g| Carb: 13g| Protein: 6g

57. Smoked Deviled Eggs

Prep Time: 15 minutes | Cooking Time: 30 minutes | Temperature: 180F| Servings: 5

Ingredients:

- 7 hard-boiled eggs, peeled
- 3 tbsp mayonnaise
- 3 tbsp chives, diced
- 1 tbsp brown mustard
- 1 tbsp apple cider vinegar
- Dash of hot sauce
- Salt and pepper
- 2 tbsp cooked bacon, crumbled
- Paprika to taste

Directions:

1. Set the temperature of the grill to 180F for 15 minutes with the lid closed.
2. Place the eggs on the grill grate and smoke the eggs for 30 minutes.
3. Remove the eggs from the grill and cool.
4. Halve the eggs and scoop the egg yolks into a zip lock bag.
5. Add all other ingredients in the zip lock bag except bacon and paprika. Mix until smooth.
6. Pipe the mixture into the egg whites, then top with bacon and paprika.
7. Serve.

NUTRITION:

Calories: 140|Fat: 12g | Carb: 1g| Protein: 6g

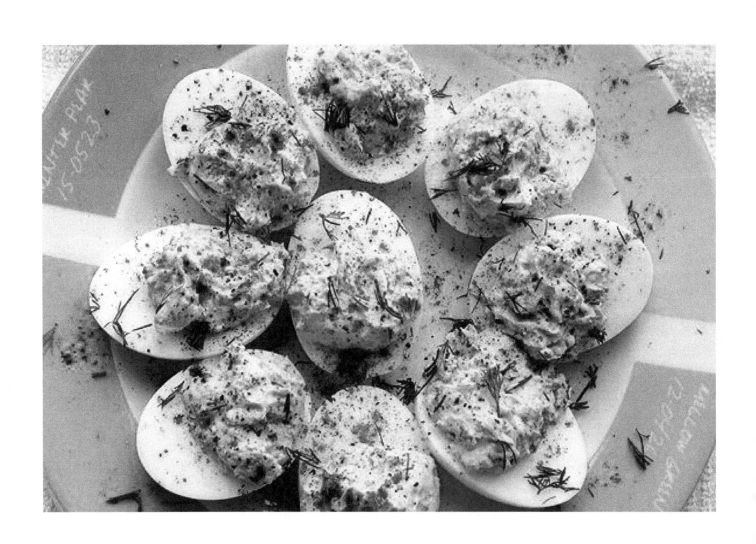

58. Smoked Asparagus

Prep Time: 5 minutes| Cooking Time: 1 hour | Temperature: 230F| Servings: 4

Ingredients:

- 1 bunch fresh asparagus, ends cut
- 2 tbsp olive oil
- Salt and pepper to taste

Directions:

1. Fire up the grill to 230F.
2. Place the asparagus in a bowl and drizzle with olive oil.
3. Season with salt and pepper.
4. Place the asparagus in a tinfoil sheet and fold the sides to create a basket.
5. Smoke the asparagus for 1 hour or until soft, turning once at the halfway mark.
6. Serve.

NUTRITION:

Calories: 43|Fat: 2g| Carb: 4g| Protein: 3g

CPSIA information can be obtained
at www.ICGtesting.com
Printed in the USA
BVHW091352110321
602276BV00014B/1295